CROHN'S DISEASE

DOCTORS TECHNIQUES FOR CURING

CROHN'S DISEASE

DR. J. SIMON

Contents

INTRODUCTION

Crohn's disease is a type of inflammatory bowel disease (IBD) that mostly affects the gastrointestinal tract. It is an ongoing ailment. The characteristic feature of this condition is inflammation, which can impact any part of the digestive system, from the mouth to the anus. Crohn's disease is a chronic condition that often goes through phases of active and remission.

Important Facts Regarding Crohn's Disease:

Inflammatory reaction

One characteristic that sets Crohn's disease apart is a persistent state of inflammation that can affect multiple layers of the intestinal wall. The inflammation may cause a variety of symptoms and effects.

Sections of the Interaction:

Crohn's disease can affect any part of the digestive system, which includes the stomach, esophagus, small and large intestines (colon). Where the inflammation appears in segments, there may be healthy tissue between the affected areas.

Warning signs:

The typical symptoms of Crohn's disease include fatigue, diarrhea, weight loss, and occasionally fever. The severity of symptoms varies from individual to person.

CHAPTER ONE

Issues

Intestinal strictures, fistulas (abnormal connections between organs), abscesses, and ulcer development are examples of complications from Crohn's disease. These problems may require surgery or other medical care.

Relapses and Remissions:

Crohn's disease is characterized by periods of active flare-ups spaced out by remissions, in which the disease's symptoms may reduce or go away.

Apart from the digestive system, joint pain, skin rashes, and ocular inflammation are possible extraintestinal symptoms of Crohn's disease.

The Constituent Autoimmune

The exact cause of Crohn's disease is still unknown, however it is believed to be the result of a complex interaction of immune system, environmental, and genetic factors. When the immune system mistakenly targets the gastrointestinal tract, inflammation ensues.

The diagnosis procedure makes use of the patient's medical history, physical examination, laboratory testing, and imaging methods (such as endoscopies and colonoscopies). Biopsies could be taken during these treatments to confirm the presence of inflammation.

Counseling:

The goals of treatment include lowering inflammation, controlling symptoms, and improving quality of life. Anti-inflammatory drugs, immunosuppressants, and biologics are among the often utilized pharmaceuticals. In certain cases, surgery may be necessary to address issues or remove the affected intestinal segments.

Individuals with Crohn's disease should work closely with gastroenterologists and other medical specialists to develop a personalized treatment strategy. Making dietary changes, changing one's lifestyle, and receiving continuous medical care are often part of a comprehensive plan for managing Crohn's disease.

Knowing What Crohn's Disease Is

Understanding Crohn's disease requires understanding its fundamental traits, causes, symptoms, diagnosis, and course of treatment. Let's take a closer look at each of the numerous aspects of Crohn's disease:

Crucial attributes:

Extended Inflammation:

One of the main characteristics of Crohn's disease is chronic inflammation of the gastrointestinal system, which can affect any part of the body, including the mouth and the anus. The inflammation often permeates the several layers of the gut wall.

Partially Involved:

Unlike some other inflammatory bowel diseases, Crohn's disease typically affects the parts of the digestive tract where healthy tissue is between the affected portions. Its "skip pattern" helps to distinguish it from conditions like ulcerative colitis.

Variations in Symptoms:

The symptoms that people with Crohn's disease encounter might vary greatly. The following are common indications and symptoms: fever, weariness, diarrhea, and stomach ache. The combination and degree of symptoms may vary over time.

Intestinal strictures, fistulas (abnormal connections between organs), abscesses, and ulcer development are examples of complications from Crohn's disease. To address these concerns, surgery or other medical procedures might be necessary.

Outside the Intestine Manifestations:

In addition to the gastrointestinal system, Crohn's disease can also cause symptoms to manifest outside of it, affecting the joints, skin, eyes, and other organs. These symptoms that are extraintestinal exacerbate the illness.

Genetic Components:

Genetic predisposition has a role in the onset of Crohn's disease. Those with a family history of IBD, especially Crohn's disease, may be at higher risk.

Immunological System Deficit:

Crohn's disease is regarded as an autoimmune disease that results in inflammation when the immune system mistakenly attacks the gastrointestinal tract. What precisely triggers this immune response is unknown.

Environmental Factors:

Environmental factors such as diet, smoking, and exposure to certain infections may contribute to the development or exacerbation of Crohn's disease in genetically predisposed individuals.

Medical History and Physical Examination:

A thorough medical history and physical examination are carried out in order to assess the symptoms' severity, duration, and any potential risk factors.

Imaging Studies:

Using imaging examinations, one may see the gastrointestinal tract, locate inflammatory regions, and take biopsy samples. Endoscopy, colonoscopy, and imaging tests (such CT or MRI) are some of these procedures.

Laboratory Tests:

Testing for anemia, inflammation, and other markers associated with Crohn's disease can be done on blood samples.

Substances:

Numerous medications, including biologics, immunosuppressants, and anti-inflammatory drugs, are used to treat Crohn's disease. The ideal medication depends on the kind and severity of the symptoms.

Modifications to Lifestyle:

Eating differently, controlling stress, and avoiding known triggers can all contribute to overall wellness and symptom relief.

Surgery:

In certain cases, surgery may be necessary to treat specific issues like fistulas or strictures, to deal with complications, or to remove damaged colon tissue.

Constant Monitoring

Regular visits to medical specialists are essential for monitoring the course of a disease, addressing emerging concerns, and modifying treatment plans as needed.

A complete comprehension of Crohn's disease requires consideration of the complex interplay among immunological, environmental, and genetic components. If Crohn's disease is correctly diagnosed and treated, patients can successfully manage their symptoms and have happy, satisfying lives.

Motives and Risk Factors

The exact cause of Crohn's disease is unknown, however it is believed to be the result of a combination of immune system, environmental, and genetic factors. There are several logical explanations and risk factors that have been identified:

1. Genetic Components:

There is a significant genetic component to Crohn's disease. An increased risk of developing Crohn's disease or other inflammatory bowel disorders (IBDs) runs in families. Crohn's disease risk has been associated with specific genetic variations, including those in the NOD2 gene.

2. Immunological System Deficit:

As an autoimmune disorder, Crohn's disease is typified by inflammation brought on by the immune system unintentionally targeting cells in the gastrointestinal tract. It is thought that a combination of genetic and environmental variables have a role in this immunological response, even though the exact reason is unknown.

3. Environmental Factors:

Certain environmental factors can cause Crohn's disease to get worse or develop in the first place. Among them are:

Smoking: Research has demonstrated that smoking is a significant risk factor for Crohn's disease and exacerbates its severity.

Food does not directly cause Crohn's disease, although there are dietary factors that can influence the disease's course and risk. There is a risk associated with consuming significant amounts of sugar and processed fats.

Microbial Exposure: In people who are susceptible to Crohn's disease, exposure to specific infections or changes in the gut microbiome may be responsible for inducing an aberrant immune response.

4. Ethnicity and Age:

Although Crohn's disease can strike at any age, it usually starts in adolescence or the early stages of adulthood. People who are Ashkenazi Jews are more likely to have Crohn's disease.

5. Place of Geographical Origin:

Compared to developing countries, Western industrialized nations have a higher prevalence of Crohn's disease. This geographical heterogeneity raises the possibility that environmental variables, including diet and lifestyle, play a part in the disease's progression.

6. Past Infections of the Gastrointestines:

According to certain research, having a history of gastrointestinal tract infections may make Crohn's disease more likely to occur. Certain vulnerable people may experience an aberrant immune response as a result of infections.

7. Contraceptives by mouth:

There is some data that points to a possible link between using oral contraceptives, or birth control pills, and a higher chance of getting Crohn's disease. To fully comprehend this correlation, more research is necessary because the relationship is complex.

It's crucial to remember that while having certain risk factors may increase the likelihood of getting Crohn's disease, not everyone who has them will end up with the illness. Likewise, Crohn's disease can strike certain people even in the absence of obvious risk factors. Understanding the etiology of Crohn's disease requires a thorough understanding of the intricate interplay between genetic and environmental variables.

Symptoms and Indications

Numerous indications and symptoms that impact the gastrointestinal system and, occasionally, other body areas might be present with Crohn's disease. Individual differences can be seen in the way symptoms present, as well as changes in the intensity of symptoms over time. Some common indications and manifestations of Crohn's disease are:

1. Pain in the abdomen:

One of the most common signs of Crohn's disease is persistent or recurrent stomach pain. The discomfort may be localized in particular locations of the abdomen and is frequently crampy.

2. Diarrhea

One common sign of Crohn's disease is chronic diarrhea. There could be frequent, loose, and watery stools, which could lead to malnutrition and dehydration.

3. Loss of Weight:

CHAPTER TWO

In those with Crohn's disease, inadvertent weight loss is frequently seen. A number of things, including decreased appetite, nutrient malabsorption, and inflammation, can cause this.

4. Weary:

Fatigue, weakness, and a generalized sense of exhaustion might result from chronic inflammation and the body's reaction to the illness.

5. Temperature spike:

Fever episodes are common in some Crohn's disease patients, particularly when there is active inflammation.

6. Bleeding in the Rectal Area:

Rectal bleeding may result from inflammation in the rectum or other areas of the gastrointestinal system. There could be blood on the toilet paper or in the feces.

7. Symptoms of Perianal:

Anal fissures, abscesses, and fistulas are among the symptoms of Crohn's disease that can affect the perianal region. Pain and discomfort may be brought on by these symptoms.

8. alterations in bowel habits

Changes in bowel habits, such as urgency, partial evacuation, and urgency of bowel movement, can occur in individuals with Crohn's disease.

9. vomiting and nauseous:

During illness flare-ups in particular, nausea and vomiting are possible. These symptoms may be exacerbated by small intestinal or stomach inflammation.

10. Joint Soreness and Edema:

Arthralgia, also referred to as joint discomfort and swelling, is a condition that some people with Crohn's disease encounter. The joints in the extremities may be impacted by these extraintestinal symptoms.

11. Skin Issues:

Skin conditions such rashes, redness, or uncomfortable nodules can be brought on by Crohn's disease. A particular type of skin problem called erythema nodosum is linked to inflammatory bowel disorders.

12. Inflammation of the eyes:

People with Crohn's disease may get uveitis or episcleritis, an inflammation of the eyes that causes redness, discomfort, and light sensitivity.

It's crucial to understand that Crohn's disease progresses in an unpredictable way, alternating between remission and periods of active symptoms, or flare-ups. Furthermore, not every person with Crohn's disease will have the same set of symptoms or degree of severity. For people with Crohn's disease, managing their symptoms and enhancing their quality of life depend heavily on an early diagnosis and adequate medical care. See a medical expert for a complete assessment and diagnosis if you think you might have Crohn's disease or if your gastrointestinal symptoms are bothersome.

Diagnosis and Assessment

A combination of medical history, physical examination, imaging scans, laboratory testing, and, in certain situations, endoscopic treatments are used to diagnose Crohn's disease. The goals of the diagnostic procedure are to evaluate the patient's symptoms, pinpoint the site and degree of inflammation, rule out other illnesses, and choose the best course of action. The following are essential elements of the diagnosis and assessment of Crohn's disease:

1. Medical History and Physical Examination:

In order to evaluate the symptoms, their duration, and any relevant risk factors, a thorough medical history is gathered. A comprehensive physical assessment, with abdominal probing, is carried out to detect indications of inflammation or problems.

2. Blood Tests:

To evaluate several markers linked to inflammation, anemia, and nutritional deficits, blood tests can be carried out. Typical blood examinations for Crohn's disease consist of:

The ESR (erythrocyte sedimentation rate) and C-reactive protein (CRP)

Tests of liver function

tests for iron, vitamin B12, and folate levels, among other nutritional deficits

3. Stool Examinations:

It is possible to get stool samples in order to look for indicators of inflammation, infectious pathogens, and blood. Stool tests offer further details on the nature of symptoms and aid in ruling out other gastrointestinal disorders.

4. Imaging Studies:

The gastrointestinal tract may be seen, and the degree of inflammation can be determined, using several imaging investigations. Common imaging methods include:

Colonoscopy: To see the lining of the gut directly, a flexible tube equipped with a camera is inserted into the colon during this operation.

Endoscopy: An upper endoscopy can be used to see inside the stomach and esophagus as well as the upper gastrointestinal tract.

Capsule endoscopy: This method involves swallowing a capsule with a camera inside of it so that the small intestine can be seen.

Computed Tomography (CT) Scan: CT scans can identify areas of inflammation, strictures, or problems and offer detailed images of the abdomen and pelvis.

When radiation exposure is a problem, magnetic resonance imaging, or MRI, can be utilized to evaluate the colon and adjacent structures.

5. autopsy

Tissue samples (biopsies) from the afflicted areas may be obtained for microscopic analysis during a colonoscopy or endoscopy. Biopsies are used to rule out other illnesses and confirm the existence of inflammation.

6. Barium Enema or Swallow:

The gastrointestinal tract may be seen with barium contrast tests. X-rays are obtained after ingesting or injecting barium into the rectum in order to detect any anomalies, strictures, or fistulas.

7. Genetic Analysis:

Assessing genetic propensity and susceptibility to Crohn's disease may involve genetic testing, especially for polymorphisms in the NOD2 gene.

8. Additional Diagnostic Pointers:

In certain instances, further examinations such capsule endoscopy, enterography, or pelvic ultrasonography could be suggested to obtain further details regarding the degree of inflammation or problems.

9. Diagnostic Differentiation:

Irritable bowel syndrome (IBS), ulcerative colitis, and infections are among the gastrointestinal disorders that share symptoms with Crohn's disease. Separating Crohn's disease from other possible causes is the goal of the diagnostic procedure.

The final diagnosis of Crohn's disease is usually established by combining information from imaging, laboratory, clinical, and histology tests. After receiving a diagnosis, people with Crohn's disease can collaborate with medical specialists to create a customized treatment plan that addresses problems, induces remission, and manages symptoms. For those with Crohn's disease to have better long-term outcomes and a higher quality of life, early diagnosis and treatments are essential.

Crohn's disease types and patterns

Different types and patterns of gastrointestinal tract involvement can be seen in Crohn's disease. Different parts of the digestive system may be affected by the condition, and the inflammation pattern may change. The following are typical forms and trends of Crohn's disease:

1. ileocolitis

The most prevalent form of Crohn's disease is ileocolitis. Both the colon (the big intestine) and the ileum the final segment of the small intestine are inflamed. Abdominal pain, diarrhea, and weight loss are possible symptoms.

2. Ileitis:

Ileitis is the name for inflammation that is restricted to the ileum, which is the small intestine's terminal segment. Symptoms of this kind of Crohn's disease include malabsorption, diarrhea, and abdominal pain.

3. Crohn's disease with gastroduodenum:

Crohn's disease can occasionally impact the duodenum, the first segment of the small intestine, and the stomach. Symptoms of this kind of Crohn's disease, called gastroduodenal Crohn's disease, include upper abdominal pain, nausea, and vomiting.

4. Jejunoileitis:

The central section of the small intestine, the jejunum, becomes inflamed when someone has jejunoileitis. Malabsorption, discomfort in the abdomen, and other symptoms are possible.

5. Colitis of Crohn's:

The large intestine (colon) is the only area of inflammation associated with Crohn's colitis. It might show up as symptoms including urgency, stomach pain, and bloody diarrhea. Crohn's disease can cause inflammation that is patchy or segmented, affecting different areas of the colon.

6. Crohn's disease in Periana:

Inflammation in the perianal area is a symptom of perianal Crohn's disease, which can cause anal fissures, abscesses, fistulas, and skin tags. These issues may result in discomfort and pain.

7. Obstructive Pattern and Strictures:

Strictures, or intestinal narrowings, may eventually arise as a result of Crohn's disease's ongoing inflammation. An obstructive pattern brought on by strictures may manifest as symptoms including bloating, vomiting, and stomach pain.

8. Exerting force on Crohn's disease:

The development of anomalous connections, or fistulas, between various gastrointestinal tract segments or between the gut and other organs is a hallmark of fistulizing Crohn's disease.

Complications from fistulas might include pus leakage and abscesses.

9. Uncertain Collitis:

The pattern of inflammation may not always match the diagnostic criteria for ulcerative colitis or Crohn's disease. This condition is known as indeterminate colitis, and it might need to be further assessed in the future.

10. Sectional Pattern:

Crohn's disease frequently shows a segmental pattern of involvement, in which healthy bowel segments are strewn in between inflammatory ones. Crohn's disease can be distinguished from illnesses such as ulcerative colitis by its skip pattern, as the former usually entails persistent inflammation.

It's critical to remember that Crohn's disease is a diverse illness, and that different people may suffer different types or patterns of symptoms. The illness can also be distinguished by intervals of acute symptoms (flare-ups) interspersed with remissions. Treatment choices and individualised management strategies may be influenced by the unique type and pattern of Crohn's disease. To suggest appropriate interventions, healthcare practitioners assess the type and extent of Crohn's disease using a combination of clinical, imaging, and endoscopic data.

The goals of Crohn's disease treatment are to lessen symptoms, bring the illness into and keep it out of remission, and enhance overall quality of life for those who have it. The kind, location, and severity of Crohn's disease, in addition to personal characteristics like age, general health, and patient preferences, all influence the therapy option. The following are some methods of treating Crohn's disease:

1. Substances:

Anti-Inflamatory Medication:

Aminosalicylates: Medications that assist reduce colon inflammation, such mesalamine, are frequently prescribed for mild to moderate instances.

Corticosteroids:

During flare-ups, a doctor may prescribe short-term usage of corticosteroids, such as prednisone, to quickly reduce inflammation. However, because of the possible adverse consequences, prolonged usage is usually discouraged.

Regulatory T cells:

Medication such as methotrexate, 6-mercaptopurine, and azathioprine can help regulate immunity and lower inflammation. When Crohn's disease is mild to severe, they are used.

In order to reduce inflammation, biologic drugs like vedolizumab, adalimumab, and infliximab target particular immune system pathways. When alternative treatments are unsuccessful or the condition is mild to severe, biologics are frequently used.

2. Symptomatic Reduction:

Antidiarrheal Drugs: Loperamide is one medication that can be used to treat diarrhea.

Pain Management: Because they can sometimes make symptoms worse, analgesics, also known as nonsteroidal anti-inflammatory medicines

(NSAIDs), are used with caution for treating pain.

3. Dietary Therapy:

Exclusive Enteral Nutrition (EEN): Depending on the situation, especially if the patient is a youngster or the illness is active, a liquid diet that meets all of their nutritional needs may be advised.

4. Surgery:

Stricture Removal: In order to treat strictures, or narrowings, in the gut that obstruct the passage of contents, surgery may be required.

Fistula Repair: Drain abscesses and fistulas can both be treated surgically.

Resection: Surgical removal (resection) of the bowel's damaged sections may be required in cases of severe disease or consequences.

5. Disease Surveillance:

Endoscopic Monitoring: To determine the degree of inflammation, keep an eye out for problems, and inform treatment choices, routine endoscopic assessments such as colonoscopies may be advised.

Imaging Studies: To assess the state of the colon and surrounding structures, periodic imaging studies, such as CT scans or MRIs, may be performed.

6. Assistive Interventions:

Dietary Adjustments: Some people discover that by recognizing and avoiding particular trigger foods, they can alleviate their symptoms. Optimizing nutrition may be possible when working with a licensed dietitian.

Stress management: Since stress can aggravate symptoms, methods like meditation, therapy, or support groups may be helpful.

7. Immunizations:

It is crucial to make sure that people with Crohn's disease are up to date on their immunizations, especially those against the flu, pneumococcal infections, and other diseases that can be avoided.

8. Tailored Care Programs:

Healthcare providers collaborate closely with patients to customize treatment regimens that are highly personalized, taking into account their individual circumstances, preferences, and reaction to therapy.

It's critical for people with Crohn's disease to communicate openly with their medical team about their symptoms, available treatments, and any concerns they may have. Consistent monitoring and follow-up appointments guarantee that the treatment plan is still effective and can be modified as necessary. Since Crohn's disease is a chronic illness, long-term management plans emphasize on general wellbeing while putting the patient in and staying in remission.

CHAPTER THREE

Dietary and lifestyle choices are very important for controlling Crohn's disease and enhancing general health. The following broad recommendations may be beneficial for people with Crohn's disease, even if individual reactions to particular diets and lifestyle modifications can vary:

Nutritional Points to Remember:

Low-Residue Food:

In flare-ups, a low-residue or low-fiber diet may help since it lessens the volume and frequency of bowel motions. This entails staying away from foods high in fiber, like whole grains, nuts, and raw fruits and vegetables.

Simple Foods to Digestion:

Choose foods that are easy to digest, such as refined grains, lean meats, and well-cooked, peeled fruits and vegetables.

Consumption of Protein:

Make sure you're getting enough protein, as it's necessary for tissue regeneration. Lean meats, poultry, fish, eggs, and dairy products are good sources of protein.

Drinking plenty of water

Drink plenty of fluids, especially water, to stay well-hydrated. Steer clear of excessive alcohol or caffeine intake since they can exacerbate dehydration.

Dairy Goods:

It's possible for some Crohn's disease patients to be lactose intolerant. To determine tolerance, try lactose-free or low-lactose dairy products.

Restrict Foods That Trigger:

Determine which foods cause symptoms and cut them back. High-fat foods, spicy foods, and some dairy products are common triggers.

Little, Regular Meals:

Larger meals may not be as taxing on the digestive system as smaller, more frequent meals spread throughout the day.

Addenda:

Take into account nutritional supplements, like vitamins and minerals, particularly if nutrient deficits are a concern. See a medical expert before beginning any supplementation.

A Look at Lifestyle:

Handling Stress:

Use stress-relieving methods including yoga, mindfulness, meditation, and deep breathing. For certain people, stress could make their symptoms worse.

Frequent Workout:

Consistently partake in mild physical activity can enhance general health and potentially boost immunity.

Sufficient Sleep:

Make obtaining enough sleep a priority in order to maintain immune system and general wellness.

Quitting Smoking:

If you smoke, think about giving it up. Smoking can make symptoms worse and is a proven risk factor for Crohn's disease.

Keeping an eye on symptoms:

Maintain a food journal to monitor the connection between dietary decisions and flare-ups of symptoms. This can assist in determining specific triggers.

Working together with the healthcare team:

Develop and modify food regimens in close collaboration with medical specialists, such as nutritionists and gastroenterologists, taking into account each person's unique requirements and reactions.

Instruction and Assistance:

Learn about Crohn's disease, how to manage it, and what resources are out there. Consult medical experts, support groups, or online forums for assistance.

It's crucial to remember that everyone reacts differently to certain foods and lifestyle adjustments. One person's solution might not be another's. Consequently, the key is a tailored strategy directed by cooperation with medical experts. Personalized dietary recommendations based on individual needs and tastes can be obtained by consulting with a licensed dietitian who specializes in gastrointestinal problems. Scheduling routine follow-up visits with medical professionals enables continuing evaluation and dietary and lifestyle modifications.

Issues and Prolonged Consequences

Crohn's disease is a chronic illness that can affect other organs as well as the gastrointestinal system and cause a number of long-term consequences. People who have Crohn's disease should be aware of possible consequences and collaborate actively with their medical team to manage and prevent them. The following are typical side symptoms and long-term consequences of Crohn's disease:

1. Strictures of the Bowel:

Prolonged intestinal inflammation can cause scar tissue to develop, which can cause strictures or narrowings. Bowel obstruction brought on by strictures can result in symptoms like bloating, vomiting, and abdominal pain.

2. Fistulas:

A fistula is an irregular opening that forms between the gut and other organs or between sections of the gastrointestinal tract. They may result in infections, pus leaks, and abscesses, among other consequences.

3. Abscesses:

Abscesses are localized collections of pus that can develop as a result of inflammation and fistula formation. Pain, swelling, and systemic symptoms can all be caused by abscesses.

4. Perianal Difficulties:

The perianal region can give rise to issues related to the perianal area, such as anal fissures, abscesses, and fistulas. These side effects could include pain, discomfort, and trouble voiding.

5. Nutritional Deficiencies and Malnutrition:

Malabsorption and chronic inflammation can cause malnourishment and shortages in vital minerals like folate, vitamin B12, and iron.

6. The disease osteoporosis

Osteoporosis risk increases with long-term use of corticosteroids, which may be administered during flare-ups and contribute to bone density loss.

7. arthritic

Arthralgia or arthritis, which include pain and inflammation in the joints, can be extraintestinal symptoms of Crohn's disease.

8. Inflammation of the eyes:

People with Crohn's disease may experience uveitis or episcleritis, an inflammation of the eyes that causes redness, discomfort, and light sensitivity.

9. Problems with the Liver:

Crohn's disease may occasionally have an impact on the liver, resulting in diseases like autoimmune hepatitis or primary sclerosing cholangitis (PSC).

10. Enhanced Colon Cancer Risk:

People who have had colon-related Crohn's disease for a long time may be more likely to get colorectal cancer. Colonoscopies for surveillance and monitoring on a regular basis are advised.

11. Effects on the mind and emotions:

Anxiety, despair, and stress are just a few of the psychological and emotional impacts of having a chronic illness like Crohn's disease. It is crucial to have support from medical experts, support groups, or mental health specialists.

12. Surgical Aftereffects:

In certain instances, surgery might be required to treat problems such strictures, fistulas, or abscesses. Infection, hemorrhage, or the formation of new strictures are among the dangers associated with surgical operations.

People with Crohn's disease should collaborate closely with their medical team to ensure proper management techniques, early detection of problems, and routine monitoring. For those with

Crohn's disease, following medication regimens, leading healthy lives, and getting help when needed all improve general wellbeing and quality of life. Scheduling routine follow-up visits with gastroenterologists and other specialists contributes to the provision of comprehensive care and early detection and treatment of the illness and any associated problems.

Emotional Health and Coping Mechanisms

Managing the psychological and emotional effects of having a chronic illness is just as important to coping with Crohn's disease as treating its physical symptoms. The following coping mechanisms and advice can help you keep your emotional health:

1. Knowledge and comprehension:

Get as much information as you can on Crohn's disease, including its signs and symptoms, available therapies, and possible side effects. You can take an active role in your care if you are aware of your illness.

2. Honest Communication

Openly discuss your symptoms, worries, and preferred course of therapy with your medical staff. Building a solid relationship with your medical professionals encourages a team-based approach to Crohn's disease management.

3. Assist Mechanism:

Create a network of family, friends, and medical professionals for support. Talk to people you can trust and who can understand and support you emotionally about your experiences and feelings.

4. Participate in Support Groups:

Joining an online or in-person support group will allow you to interact with other people who suffer from Crohn's disease. Feelings of loneliness can be lessened and a sense of community can be created by sharing experiences with people going through comparable difficulties.

5. Support for Mental Health:

To address the emotional difficulties, worry, or sadness brought on by having a chronic illness, think about getting help from mental health specialists like psychologists or counselors.

6. Handling Stress:

Use stress-relieving methods including yoga, mindfulness, meditation, and deep breathing. Stress management is crucial since it affects one's mental and physical health.

7. Establish sensible objectives:

Set attainable objectives for yourself that account for your current state of health and energy. To help prevent feeling overwhelmed, divide more complex jobs into smaller, more doable segments.

8. Sustain an optimistic attitude:

Pay attention to the areas of your life that you have control over and the proactive measures you can take to take care of your health. Develop an optimistic outlook to improve resilience.

9. Create a Schedule:

Establishing a routine can help people feel stable and predictable, which is consoling in uncertain times. Prioritize your well-being by incorporating self-care activities into your daily routine.

10. Use Creativity to Express Yourself:

Take part in artistic, literary, or musical endeavors that provide you the opportunity to express yourself. Having a creative outlet can help you process your feelings and be therapeutic.

11. Have Self-Compassion:

Recognize that managing a chronic illness such as Crohn's disease might provide difficulties. Even if your development is small, recognize it and have patience with yourself.

12. Keep Up With Available Treatments:

Keep up with developments in the care of Crohn's disease and share any new choices you have with your medical team. You may feel more optimistic about the future if you are informed of new treatments.

13. Make a fun and relaxing plan:

Include enjoyable and relaxing activities in your daily routine. Make happy moments a priority, whether that means taking a break, engaging in hobbies, or spending time with loved ones.

CHAPTER FOUR

Remind yourself that it's acceptable to prioritize your mental and emotional health and to ask for assistance when necessary. Crohn's disease can be difficult to manage, but with the correct help and coping mechanisms, people can live happy, productive lives with their disease.

Family Planning and Pregnancy

For those with Crohn's disease, pregnancy and family planning concerns include cautious management of the illness to guarantee the health of the parent and the unborn child. The following are some essential ideas and things to think about:

1. Planning Before Conception:

See your healthcare team prior to conception if you have Crohn's disease and are thinking about getting pregnant. Planning ahead of time for pregnancy enables a thorough evaluation of your health and the best possible treatment plan.

2. Review of Medication:

Discuss your present drug schedule with your obstetrician and gastroenterologist. While certain Crohn's disease treatments may be safe to continue taking during pregnancy, others may need to be changed or stopped.

3. Control of Disease:

Prior to making an attempt at conception, strive for and maintain illness remission. Pregnancy problems are more likely to occur when there is active inflammation. To monitor disease activity and make drug adjustments, collaborate closely with your healthcare team.

4. Supplementing with Folate:

Start taking folic acid supplements prior to getting pregnant and keep taking them all the way through. In a developing fetus, folic acid helps prevent neural tube problems.

5. Frequent Prenatal Care:

Make an appointment for routine prenatal examinations with an obstetrician who specializes in handling high-risk pregnancies. In the event of any difficulties, close observation enables early discovery and intervention.

6. Diet and Nutrition:

Keep up a healthy, well-balanced diet to promote both your and your baby's wellbeing. To address specific dietary needs, particularly if malabsorption or nutrient deficiencies are a concern, collaborate with a registered dietitian.

7. Keeping an eye out for complications

Crohn's disease patients may be more susceptible to gestational diabetes, low birth weight, and preterm birth, among other pregnancy complications. Frequent observation can aid in identifying and handling these problems.

8. Considerations for Breastfeeding:

Talk to your healthcare team about your breastfeeding plans. While some Crohn's disease medications can be taken while nursing, others might need to be adjusted.

9. Cooperative Healthcare:

Make sure that your obstetrician and gastroenterologist are working together and communicating openly. To maximize care, a multidisciplinary strategy involving both specialists is necessary.

10. Customized Method:

Acknowledge that every pregnancy is different and that different people may experience different effects from Crohn's disease. It is essential to provide care that is tailored to you and takes into consideration your unique health needs and circumstances.

11. Psychological Assistance:

Ask your family, friends, and medical team for emotional support. Being pregnant can cause a range of emotions, so it can be helpful to surround yourself with supportive people.

12. Taking Medication Usage Into Account:

While some Crohn's disease medications can be taken during pregnancy, others might need to be changed or stopped. To make well-informed decisions, talk to your healthcare team about the advantages and disadvantages of prescription drugs.

Not to mention, managing Crohn's disease while pregnant necessitates cooperation between the patient, gastroenterologist, and obstetrician.

Many people with Crohn's disease are able to have successful pregnancies and healthy babies with proper planning and supervision. For personalized advice based on your unique health status and circumstances, always consult your healthcare team.

New Research and Treatments

Since my last knowledge update in January 2022, advances in the field of Crohn's disease have prompted the investigation of new treatment modalities and developing therapies. It's crucial to remember that advances in medical research happen frequently, and since my last update, there might have been more advancements or fresh discoveries. The following are some areas of Crohn's disease research and emerging therapies:

1. Bio-based Treatments:

The creation of novel biologic medications that specifically target inflammatory pathways is the main focus of ongoing research. The purpose of these medications is to give those who might not react well to current biologics more options.

2. JAK Blockers:

A class of medications known as janus kinase (JAK) inhibitors targets the JAK-STAT signaling pathway, which is implicated in inflammation. JAK inhibitors are an oral treatment option for Crohn's disease; research is ongoing to evaluate their safety and efficacy.

3. Modulators of Sphingosine-1-Phosphate Receptors:

The potential of medications like ozanimod, which target sphingosine-1-phosphate receptors, to treat inflammatory bowel diseases like Crohn's disease is being studied. These medications alter immune reactions.

4. Research on the Gut Microbiome:

The role of the gut microbiome in Crohn's disease is still being investigated. Knowing how the immune system and the microbiome interact could result in the development of novel therapeutic strategies, such as fecal microbiota transplantation (FMT) or the use of probiotics.

5. Precision Health Care:

The goal of precision medicine advancements is to customize care according to each patient's unique genetic and molecular profile. This individualized approach could result in more focused and effective Crohn's disease treatments.

6. Stem Cell Utilization:

Researchers are looking into stem cell therapy as a possible Crohn's disease treatment. The objective is to modify the immune system and repair damaged tissues using stem cells.

7. Intelligent artificial systems (AI):

Large datasets, including genetic and patient data, are being analyzed using AI and machine learning algorithms to find trends and forecast treatment outcomes. This method could lead to more individualized and successful treatment plans.

8. Nanomedicine:

Drug delivery methods based on nanoparticles are being investigated for specific drug delivery to gastrointestinal tract inflammation. This strategy may reduce side effects while increasing medication efficacy.

9. Therapy for Immune Modulation:

Immune modulation therapies, which seek to more precisely control the immune response, are still being researched. Examining novel immunomodulatory substances and pathways is part of this.

10. Patient-Reported Results and Life Quality:

Research is aimed at determining how Crohn's disease affects the quality of life of its sufferers. In order to inform holistic treatment approaches, this includes research on psychosocial aspects, mental health, and patient-reported outcomes.

People who have Crohn's disease should be aware of new developments in the field and their treatment options. For those who want to help advance the field, taking part in clinical trials might be an option. New treatment options may become available as research advances, giving people with Crohn's disease hope for better outcomes and a higher quality of life. Seeking advice from experts and medical professionals is still essential for receiving individualized and current information about managing Crohn's disease.

CONCLUSION

To sum up, Crohn's disease is a chronic inflammatory bowel disease that is complex and has a substantial impact on the lives of those who have it. Crohn's disease, which is characterized by gastrointestinal tract inflammation, can cause a variety of symptoms, difficulties, and complications.

Over time, our understanding of Crohn's disease has changed, and new discoveries in diagnosis, treatment, and management techniques have been made possible by this research. The field is making progress in a number of areas, including the development of biologic therapies, the investigation of novel treatment approaches, and a deeper understanding of the gut microbiome.

A multidisciplinary strategy involving gastroenterologists, medical professionals, and support systems is necessary to manage Crohn's disease. Individualized treatment plans are common, taking into account the patient's general health, the location of the disease, and its severity.

Although there isn't a cure for Crohn's disease, there are treatments that can help people with the illness live better lives by reducing symptoms, achieving and maintaining remission, and improving their quality of life. A holistic approach to care includes dietary adjustments, emotional stability, and lifestyle adjustments.

People who have Crohn's disease are advised to learn about new treatments, engage in conversations with their medical team, and look into support systems. Future improvements in treatments and results can be hoped for as long as research continues to make progress.

In the end, a proactive and cooperative strategy along with continuing medical research helps to further our understanding of this complicated condition and improve the lives of those who suffer from Crohn's disease.

THE END

www.ingramcontent.com/pod-product-compliance
Lightning Source LLC
Chambersburg PA
CBHW050745260726
48661CB00001B/429